Lose Weight without Hunger!

The secret to achieving permanent weight loss

Janet L Black, RN, FNP, MSN, MPH

Peaceful Heart Press
Candler, North Carolina

Table of Contents

Introduction

Have you been on a series of diets only to gain the weight back every time (and sometimes more than you lost)? Do you find yourself feeling hungry and irritable, thinking about food all the time and wanting the diet to be over with?

There a lot of diets out there and most of them will result in weight loss, if you can stay on them. But sooner or later, you go off the diet and rapidly regain the weight. Some of the diets are not healthy to stay on long-term and are designed for quick weight loss but not permanent weight loss. Yo-yo dieting where you lose fat and muscle and then gain back mostly fat, are worse than doing nothing. You need to get off the rollercoaster.

I've been where you are and through years of trial and error plus reading everything about dieting that I came across in the medical literature as well as books and articles for the layman, I finally found a way to lose weight and feel good at the same time. I want to share that with you.

Let me tell you a little about my history. For most of my life, I was at a normal weight. I weighed a few pounds more than I wanted and occasionally my weight would go up a little, I would cut back on eating and it would go back to my usual weight without too much effort. I did a fair amount of diet counseling and even ran a few weight loss groups. I used what I had been taught, that is, a diet with plenty of whole grains and very low in fat. I was great at creating personalized exchange plan diets for people. Unfortunately, most of my patients did not have long term success.

Then I had a couple of incidents occur within months of each other that caused me to put on weight. One of these was a car accident that resulted in daily pain for months. I quit exercising and started eating comfort foods, which for me were foods with sugar. I knew what I should eat but just couldn't seem to do that. I put on about 20 or 30 pounds (this was quite a while ago and I'm not sure just how much I gained). At any rate, I was over the range of normal for the first time in my life. Someone suggested a doctor-supervised liquid protein fast as a way of getting rid of the excess weight quickly. So I tried it and it worked. The pounds practically fell off and I dropped to

15 pounds below my usual weight so that I was in the lower part of the normal range for my height. I was thin and felt very attractive. I got lots of compliments from men about how good I looked and for me, this triggered some very uncomfortable feelings and brought up memories of childhood abuse.

When I went off the liquid protein shakes and re-introduced food into my diet, not only was my body wanting to gain because of the starvation diet but mentally, I needed to feel safe. I ended up gaining over 100 pounds and was obese for the first time in my life. I worked very hard on dealing with the childhood issues and recovered from that but the weight didn't go away.

I tried the traditional sort of diets such as exchange plans, shakes and potions. I read books and articles. I did low-carb, low fat and vegan diets and while some of these (especially the low-carb diets) resulted in some weight loss, I couldn't stick with them and always gained the weight back.

I was a healthcare professional telling people they needed to lose weight and yet, I couldn't do it. Eventually, I figured out that the horrible gastrointestinal problems I was having were a result of soy and removed that from my diet. I tried elimination diets but couldn't really tell if any other specific foods were causing problems. I had become diabetic, which did not come as a surprise.

I kept reading everything I could get my hands on about weight loss and learned a lot about food and how it is produced in this country. I gradually started changing some of my eating habits to avoid some of the additives and pesticides. I knew sugar was a problem for me and that it triggered overeating.   I realized that I needed to make a change and that it needed to be permanent. Quick fix crash diets just made the problem worse. This book is a result of what I learned and what worked. I lost at least 50 pounds the first year and for the first time ever, had no desire to go back to my former eating habits. I have continued to slowly lose weight and my goal is in sight. My husband is concerned that I'm going to be too thin if I don't quit losing but I will stay in the normal range. It is great to buy regular clothing and to have more energy. I haven't felt this good in years. I have normal blood sugar.

I want to share my information with others and whether you just want to drop a few pounds or you want to lose a lot or maybe you just want to eat healthier, you will understand more about food and how it affects you as well as looking at the mental aspects of weight loss. If you aren't overweight, I hope you will develop some empathy for those who are because it is such a big problem and it really is a challenge to become thin. For me, it has gone from being a struggle to being effortless. I want the same for you!

Diets Don't Work

Actually, they do work...temporarily. The problem with our concept of dieting is that one "goes on a diet" with the understanding that, after losing some weight, one will then go off the diet. Dieting is not a manner of living for most of us but a quick fix. Ours is a culture of looking for the fast and easy way. Weight loss does not lend itself to this type of approach. That is why it is one of the most difficult problems to treat. And there is an entire "diet industry" out there devoted to selling you all kinds of special foods, pills, potions and programs. Take a look around you and you will see all kinds of products for sale while rates of obesity and overweight continue to climb. The diet industry as a whole is not dedicated to helping people successfully lose weight and keep it off so much as they are devoted to making lots of money.

At the time I'm writing this, more than two-thirds of Americans are overweight and as other countries adopt an Americanized lifestyle, they see similar results.

Overweight is defined as a body mass index (BMI) of 25 or more. I'll explain BMI in a minute. Of those who are overweight, those who have a BMI of 30 or more are categorized as obese. About 35% of people in the U.S. are considered obese. The BMI uses height and weight to estimate the amount of body fat. Since it is not measuring body fat directly, it can be inaccurate with some people such as athletes who have a lot of muscle and will overestimate their amount of body fat. In older people who have lost muscle, it can underestimate the amount of fat. Underwater weighing is most the accurate way to determine the amount of body fat but is not feasible for most of us. BMI gives us an approximation. The easiest way to figure out your BMI is to use a chart such as the one below. This chart doesn't include all heights and weights and if you find you are not on the chart, you can look up a more detailed one for more specific information but for most of us, this gives us a general idea.

To use the chart, find your height in inches, go across the table to find your weight in pounds, then look at the number at the top of that column. That is your BMI.

If your BMI is below 18.5, you are underweight.

If your BMI is between 18.5 and 24.9, your weight is normal.

If your BMI is between 25 and 29.9, you are overweight.

If your BMI is between 30 and 39.9, you are obese.

If your BMI is over 40, you are extremely obese.

You can also use the chart to see what your weight should be by looking at the weights for your height that are between 18.5 and 24.9. Before starting to lose weight, you want to determine how you are doing now and then have a realistic goal for a normal weight.

BMI	19	20	22	24	25	26	28	30	32	34	36	38	40
Ht					Wt	in	lbs						
58	91	96	105	115	119	124	134	143	153	162	172	181	191
59	94	99	109	119	124	128	138	148	158	168	178	188	198
60	97	102	112	123	128	133	143	153	163	174	184	194	204
61	100	106	116	127	132	137	148	158	169	180	190	201	211
62	104	109	120	131	136	142	153	164	175	186	196	207	218
63	107	113	124	135	141	146	158	169	180	191	203	214	225
64	110	116	128	140	145	151	163	174	186	197	209	221	232
65	114	120	132	144	150	156	168	180	192	204	216	228	240
66	118	124	136	148	155	161	173	186	198	210	223	235	247
67	121	127	140	153	159	166	178	191	204	217	230	242	255
68	125	131	144	158	164	171	184	197	210	223	236	249	262
69	128	135	149	162	169	176	189	203	216	230	243	257	270
70	132	139	153	167	174	181	195	209	222	236	250	264	278
71	136	143	157	172	179	186	200	215	229	243	257	272	286
72	140	147	162	177	184	191	206	221	235	250	265	279	294
73	144	151	166	182	189	197	212	227	242	257	272	288	302
74	148	155	171	186	194	202	218	233	249	264	280	295	311
75	152	160	176	192	200	208	224	240	256	272	287	303	319
76	156	164	180	197	205	213	230	246	263	279	295	312	328

Source: Adapted from Clinical Guidelines on the Identification, Evaluation, and Treatment of Overweight and Obesity in Adults: The Evidence Report.

Some other ways to look at your weight are to consider where the fat is located. Abdominal fat puts you at greater risk for obesity related diseases. Health risks associated with being overweight or obese include coronary heart disease, high blood pressure, stroke, type 2 diabetes, abnormal blood fats, metabolic syndrome, cancer, osteoarthritis, sleep apnea, reproductive problems and gallstones.

Besides the health risks, being overweight or obese is just not fun. It is harder to move around, it is harder to find flattering clothes that fit, you don't like the way you look and you can even be discriminated against. You know that you don't like being fat, you want to be healthier and you have a good idea how much you would like to eventually lose. Next, let's look at whether you are ready to lose weight.

Readiness to Lose Weight

Before attempting to lose weight, it is good to be aware of your current habits, preferences and any problems that might get in your way. If you have been on diets in the past, can you identify where you had problems and what might have caused you to fail?

Just because we consciously want to lost weight, doesn't mean that we don't have subconscious reasons that can prevent us from losing. Until you are able to identify and do something about those subconscious beliefs, you are going to sabotage your efforts to lose weight. If you have tried lots of diets with limited success and end up gaining the weight back, you may have reasons that you are unaware of for maintaining that extra weight.

There can also be physical reasons that make it hard for you to lose weight and you want to make sure you rule out any physical problems before you get started. We tend to want to blame our "sluggish metabolism" or anything else we can think of and, occasionally, this can be an underlying problem. It is always a good idea to see your healthcare provider periodically to make sure you don't have a problem such as an underactive thyroid. The thyroid is the gland that controls your metabolism so if it is not producing enough thyroid hormone, you tend to gain weight, feel cold all the time, have dry skin and hair, have slowed reflexes etc. Your health care provider can do blood tests to check for underlying problems such as this.

Depression is another problem that can affect your appetite and ability to sleep, which in turn, can affect your weight. If you find yourself feeling unusually sad, with little energy and sleeping too much or too little, you might want to talk to your health care provider about this. You will want to have your vitamin D level and your thyroid checked before considering a diagnosis of depression since low vitamin D and an underactive thyroid can both cause similar symptoms. If you are experiencing some mild depression, I don't advocate that you start an antidepressant since they have many side effects, including weight gain. We will talk about natural ways to treat this later and only if those are ineffective, should you consider prescription medication. If you are having thoughts of suicide, you need to contact your provider right away and get help.

Once you have ruled out any physical causes, then you can look for emotional reasons. When you think about being at a normal weight, is there anything that triggers any uncomfortable feelings? What could happen? Might you attract unwanted attention from the opposite sex (or the same sex, depending on your sexual orientation)? Might your friends abandon you? Might others have different expectations of you? Could others expect you to do more, or do things that are difficult for you? What are some of the advantages of being "bigger"?

A nutritionist friend of mine once asked a group of overweight ladies she was working with about the advantages of being heavy and was surprised to hear them say how they were better organized so that they could do things without moving around as much. By the time they listed advantages of being heavy, including eating what they wanted and being like their heavy friends, she could see why they weren't having any success in losing weight. Research has shown that you are more likely to be overweight if the people you spend time with are overweight so you might want to find some slim friends to hang out with or see if you can interest your heavy friends in making changes.

Do you associate being larger with being stronger? This is probably more important to men. Where you ever bullied by a bigger kid? You could have decided then that it was better to be larger. Looking back at times you were thinner and times that you gained weight may give you some insights as to thoughts you have had and interpretations of past events that led you to believe that you are better off being heavier. As children, we don't think logically and may misinterpret events. What we decide about the meaning of things in our lives determines thoughts and beliefs that can be held in the subconscious mind where they affect our current behavior without our even being aware. We can sabotage our efforts to lose weight as a result of these beliefs and not realize we are doing it.

Having the right mind-set plays a big part in whether you are successful in losing weight. Do you see yourself as a slender person who eats healthy foods and is active? Being able to visualize yourself this way is important for your success. Your body reflects your self-image. If you picture yourself as overweight and unable to lose the weight, that is what you will get. Take a moment and close your eyes. See yourself as a thin and active person. How do you feel? What is your life like? Is this easy or difficult for you to do?

Another thing to think about is your willingness to delay gratification. What I'm talking about here is whether you can give up the pleasure of that cookie right now because it is not a good choice for your long-term success at losing weight. When you have a choice between something you want right now and being willing to give that up if it is in conflict with your long range plans, how successful are you? How badly do you want to succeed? The ability to delay gratification matters in other areas of your life too. When you are in school, you have to make choices between studying and hanging out with friends. When you are working, you have to make choices about what you are going to do during your workday. Do you do the minimum and then spend time chatting with co-workers or do you go the extra mile to do the best work you can? Do you take the time away from doing things for yourself to do thoughtful things for friends and family?

It is hard to be successful at losing weight if you can't delay gratification. All day long you are faced with choices about what you are going to do and what you are going to eat. You are going to have to want to lose weight badly enough that you will focus on your goal and recognize that tempting foods that appear in your life aren't that important in the overall scheme of things. Eating healthy has to be a bigger priority than pie, cake, cookies, bread or whatever your favorite foods are. I'm not saying that you might not be eating those things but you won't be mindlessly consuming large quantities of them, just because they are available.

Do you have a problem with emotional hunger? What I mean is that when you have something happen that makes you sad, angry, depressed or even excited, do you head for a snack? Do you eat "comfort foods" to make yourself feel better? Usually comfort foods are those high in sugar, starch or fat. If you eat for emotional reasons, I'm sure you can identify what foods you want at those times. For me, cookies were my favorite, especially homemade chocolate chip cookies.

Eating, especially eating comfort foods, can make you feel better temporarily because it triggers the release of dopamine, a chemical in your brain. Dopamine is a neurotransmitter in your brain that makes it possible for certain neurons to send impulses to other neurons. It is associated with pleasure so anything that makes you feel good, triggers the release of dopamine. Cocaine and other drugs that make you feel good trigger the release of lots of dopamine and this is why people want to take them. In order to control our eating, we have to find more effective ways of dealing with our feelings and to make ourselves feel good. A couple of things that I've found to be effective are meditation and gratitude. First thing in the morning, I do about 15 minutes of meditation and I journal which includes writing down things that I am grateful for. This gets the day off to a good start and I tend to be happier all day.

Yesterday was not a good day for me. I saw the dentist and was told that I needed expensive dental treatment. While my mood was affected, it never even occurred to me to eat as a result. I can't say for sure if this is a result of habit or learning new ways of coping but looking back at yesterday, I ate in response to physical hunger, not emotional hunger. Since I did eat in response to emotions in the past, it is very possible to change this behavior. We will talk more about this later.

Some other things to think about are how aware are you of what you are eating? Do you find yourself eating without even thinking about it? For some people, writing down everything they eat helps with this. Personally, I know this is something that I will not do over a long period, although I can do it for brief periods such as for a week. The research shows that it does help people lose weight successfully. My experience with counseling others for weight loss is that people who will stick to keeping a diet diary do tend to comply more with a diet. However, what we are engaging in here is not a diet but a way of life. If you are like me, you aren't going to write down what you eat for the rest of your life. You might, however, want to do it briefly, just to make you more aware of your eating. This can be a good thing to do before you even make any changes so that you know what habits you have now.

Another thing that helps people is to pay more attention while they are eating. Avoid distractions like watching TV or reading and instead, pay attention to the taste of the food. Notice the texture and the smell. Sit at the table, rather than grabbing something on the run. Slow down your eating and chew your food well. Don't eat while you are driving. These things will all increase the pleasure you get from what you are eating. If you have ever eaten something without being aware and been surprised that the food was gone, this will help you.

Another advantage of paying attention and slowing down the process of eating is that you get a chance to notice when you are full. I have worked at jobs where lunch was a rushed affair and learned to eat quickly. I had to learn to slow down and that gives me a chance to be aware that I am full before I overeat.

Do you like lots of structure such as specific meal plans for what you are going to eat all week? Or would you rather decide what you want just before you fix it? It is good to be aware of your preferences. I have some idea of what I am going to have during the week according to what I get at the store but don't decide what I'm going to eat for a particular meal on most days until shortly before the time to prepare it. For example, I had decided that I wanted to make lasagna this week and bought the ingredients but didn't know what day I would make it. Yesterday, I had plenty of time to prepare and cook it so that was the day I made it. If you like to plan your meals, you will want to write out a plan and prepare your shopping list accordingly. If you are more like me, you will want to have plenty of things to prepare healthy meals and just make sure that you have everything available for whatever you decide to make. I see what is on special at the store that week and may plan meals accordingly.

Do the people around you support your weight loss? Have you had family or friends sabotage your efforts to lose weight in the past? Sometimes your family and friends don't feel comfortable with you changing. Your partner might not want you to look more attractive to others. Your friends might want you to be more like them, especially if part of your relationship is involved with eating. Family can be the same way. They are used to you the way you are and behaving the way you do now. They might not even be aware that they are sabotaging your efforts. If you are going to be able to resist sabotage, you need to understand when it is happening.

Everything in this chapter is designed to help you raise your awareness before you start making any changes and to deal with any problems that are going to prevent you from being successful. You don't want to make changes until you are ready and prepared to deal with issues that are going to arise.

What is Hunger?

Hunger is a result of your blood sugar being low. When we eat, food is absorbed from our intestines. The sugars and starches we eat are broken down into glucose, the form of sugar that your body uses for energy. This is carried through the body in your blood to provide energy for all of the cells in your body. When your blood sugar increases as a result of eating, your pancreas, an organ near the stomach, puts out a hormone into the blood stream called insulin. I'm sure you have heard of this as the stuff that diabetics give themselves by injection to bring their blood sugar down. The right amount of insulin brings the blood sugar down into a normal range. It does this by moving the blood glucose out of the blood stream and into the cells in your body so they can use it for energy.

If there is more glucose than what is needed for the body's current energy needs, the rest is converted into fat and stored. If there is too much insulin, either from the pancreas or from an injection, the blood sugar drops too much so that you are hungry and depending on how low it goes, you may experience mental confusion, shakiness, or even pass out. Because the glucose was moved from the blood stream to the cells, there is more likely to be an excess of it in the cells that will be stored as fat. So, in short, **too much insulin makes you hungry and fat**.

So what causes your body to put out too much insulin? This is a result of your blood sugar rising very rapidly. This occurs when you eat sugar or foods that convert quickly to sugar. So, you eat candy, your blood sugar spikes, your pancreas responds by releasing lots of insulin, causing your blood sugar to crash and then you are hungry again. This causes you to eat again and if you choose more quickly digested food, the cycle repeats. You will hear people say that diabetes is not caused by eating too much sugar but can you see how eating sugar and other quickly digested sweet and starchy foods can cause excess insulin output and fat storage? Being overweight is definitely a risk factor for type 2 diabetes, the common type that occurs in adults.

To control hunger, our goal is to prevent those spikes by eating foods that digest more slowly and will slow the rise of blood sugar so that the pancreas will release a smaller amount of insulin. Proteins and fats digest slowly and do not cause blood sugar spikes. Fiber is indigestible stuff found in plant foods that slows the absorption of food to help prevent blood sugar spikes. By incorporating more of these foods into each meal or snack, we can avoid blood sugar crashes with the resulting hunger and food cravings.

For many people, sugar can seem like an addiction. The more of it you eat, the more you want. By significantly reducing the amount of sugar in the diet, you can reduce food cravings and actually learn to be more sensitive to the taste of sweets so that you don't want excessively sweet foods. They will taste too sweet.

I'm not saying that you can never eat anything sweet but you will want to be very cautious about the use of sugar. I also don't recommend artificially sweetened foods as most of the sweeteners used are not that healthy. Aspartame, also known as Equal, Nutrasweet and Amino Sweet, and Sucrolose, found in Splenda, are the two most popular artificial sweeteners and they have both been found to have adverse effects on the body and to cause weight gain. I will give you more information in the chapter on sweeteners.

You may have heard about other hormones that affect weight. Leptin is a hormone that suppresses appetite that has been in the news. Ghrelin is another hormone associated with eating and stimulates the appetite. There is research going on to see if there is a way to use our knowledge of these hormones in helping people lose weight. Cortisol is a hormone produced by the adrenal cortex that also has an effect on weight. It becomes elevated during stress. We will talk more about what we can do to affect these hormones in the chapter on lifestyle changes. Next let's talk about how your body responds to different foods.

The Glycemic Index and Glycemic Load

The glycemic index is a way of rating foods as to how they affect blood sugar. Foods high on the glycemic index raise blood glucose more than those that are low. The closer something is to pure glucose, the faster it will be absorbed and raise blood sugar. If you are trying to prevent blood sugar spikes, your goal is to eat as low on the glycemic index as possible. Glycemic Load is similar but is a measurement of the total amount of carbohydrates (sugars and starches) in the food times the glycemic index. So, it takes into account the serving size. Below is a chart showing the glycemic index and load for some common foods. The serving sizes are given in grams and there are about 28 grams in an ounce.

Glycemic index and glycemic load for 100+ foods

FOOD	Glycemic index (glucose = 100)	Serving size (grams)	Glycemic load per serving
BAKERY PRODUCTS AND BREADS			
Banana cake, made with sugar	47	60	14
Banana cake, made without	55	60	12

sugar			
Sponge cake, plain	46	63	17
Vanilla cake made from packet mix with vanilla frosting (Betty Crocker)	42	111	24
Apple, made with sugar	44	60	13
Apple, made without sugar	48	60	9
Waffles, Aunt Jemima (Quaker Oats)	76	35	10
Bagel, white, frozen	72	70	25
Baguette, white, plain	95	30	15
Coarse barley bread, 75-80% kernels, average	34	30	7
Hamburger bun	61	30	9
Kaiser roll	73	30	12
Pumpernickel bread	56	30	7
50% cracked wheat kernel bread	58	30	12
White wheat flour bread	71	30	10
Wonder™ bread, average	73	30	10
Whole wheat bread, average	71	30	9
100% Whole Grain™ bread (Natural Ovens)	51	30	7
Pita bread, white	68	30	10
Corn tortilla	52	50	12
Wheat tortilla	30	50	8
BEVERAGES			
Coca Cola®, average	63	250 mL	16
Fanta®, orange soft drink	68	250 mL	23
Apple juice, unsweetened, average	44	250 mL	30
Cranberry juice cocktail (Ocean Spray®)	68	250 mL	24

Gatorade	78	250 mL	12
Orange juice, unsweetened	50	250 mL	12
Tomato juice, canned	38	250 mL	4
BREAKFAST CEREALS AND RELATED PRODUCTS			
All-Bran™, average	55	30	12
Coco Pops™, average	77	30	20
Cornflakes™, average	93	30	23
Cream of Wheat™ (Nabisco)	66	250	17
Cream of Wheat™, Instant (Nabisco)	74	250	22
Grapenuts™, average	75	30	16
Muesli, average	66	30	16
Oatmeal, average	55	250	13
Instant oatmeal, average	83	250	30
Puffed wheat, average	80	30	17
Raisin Bran™ (Kellogg's)	61	30	12
Special K™ (Kellogg's)	69	30	14
GRAINS			
Pearled barley, average	28	150	12
Sweet corn on the cob, average	60	150	20
Couscous, average	65	150	9
Quinoa	53	150	13
White rice, average	89	150	43
Quick cooking white basmati	67	150	28
Brown rice, average	50	150	16
Converted, white rice (Uncle Ben's®)	38	150	14
Whole wheat kernels, average	30	50	11
Bulgur, average	48	150	12
COOKIES AND CRACKERS			

Graham crackers	74	25	14
Vanilla wafers	77	25	14
Shortbread	64	25	10
Rice cakes, average	82	25	17
Rye crisps, average	64	25	11
Soda crackers	74	25	12
DAIRY PRODUCTS AND ALTERNATIVES			
Ice cream, regular	57	50	6
Ice cream, premium	38	50	3
Milk, full fat	41	250mL	5
Milk, skim	32	250 mL	4
Reduced-fat yogurt with fruit, average	33	200	11
FRUITS			
Apple, average	39	120	6
Banana, ripe	62	120	16
Dates, dried	42	60	18
Grapefruit	25	120	3
Grapes, average	59	120	11
Orange, average	40	120	4
Peach, average	42	120	5
Peach, canned in light syrup	40	120	5
Pear, average	38	120	4
Pear, canned in pear juice	43	120	5
Prunes, pitted	29	60	10
Raisins	64	60	28
Watermelon	72	120	4
BEANS AND NUTS			
Baked beans, average	40	150	6
Blackeye peas, average	33	150	10
Black beans	30	150	7

Chickpeas, average	10	150	3
Chickpeas, canned in brine	38	150	9
Navy beans, average	31	150	9
Kidney beans, average	29	150	7
Lentils, average	29	150	5
Soy beans, average	15	150	1
Cashews, salted	27	50	3
Peanuts, average	7	50	0
PASTA and NOODLES			
Fettucini, average	32	180	15
Macaroni, average	47	180	23
Macaroni and Cheese (Kraft)	64	180	32
Spaghetti, white, boiled, average	46	180	22
Spaghetti, white, boiled 20 min, average	58	180	26
Spaghetti, wholemeal, boiled, average	42	180	17
SNACK FOODS			
Corn chips, plain, salted, average	42	50	11
Fruit Roll-Ups®	99	30	24
M & M's®, peanut	33	30	6
Microwave popcorn, plain, average	55	20	6
Potato chips, average	51	50	12
Pretzels, oven-baked	83	30	16
Snickers Bar®	51	60	18
VEGETABLES			
Green peas, average	51	80	4
Carrots, average	35	80	2
Parsnips	52	80	4

Baked russet potato, average	111	150	33
Boiled white potato, average	82	150	21
Instant mashed potato, average	87	150	17
Sweet potato, average	70	150	22
Yam, average	54	150	20
MISCELLANEOUS			
Hummus (chickpea salad dip)	6	30	0
Chicken nuggets, frozen, reheated in microwave oven 5 min	46	100	7
Pizza, plain baked dough, served with parmesan cheese and tomato sauce	80	100	22
Pizza, Super Supreme (Pizza Hut)	36	100	9
Honey, average	61	25	12

The complete list of the glycemic index and glycemic load for more than 1,000 foods can be found in the article "International tables of glycemic index and glycemic load values: 2008" by Fiona S. Atkinson, Kaye Foster-Powell, and Jennie C. Brand-Miller in the December 2008 issue of **Diabetes Care**, Vol. 31, number 12, pages 2281-2283.

An earlier version of this table appeared here: "**International tables of glycemic index and glycemic load values: 2002**," by Kaye Foster-Powell, Susanna H.A. Holt, and Janette C. Brand-Miller in the July 2002 American Journal of Clinical Nutrition, Vol. 62, pages 5–56.

In general, whole foods are going to be lower than more processed foods. Tropical fruits such as bananas and pineapple tend to be higher. You will notice that watermelon's glycemic index is high but the glycemic load is low due to the water and fiber found in it. Dried fruits are very dense and therefore, high. Most vegetables, other than the starchy ones like potatoes and corn, are low on the glycemic index and load.

Can you eat foods that are high on the glycemic index and still lose weight? Yes, but the secret is to eat small amounts mixed with other foods that are low. You will notice that you did not see eggs, meat, cheese or fats on the list. That is because they don't raise blood sugar significantly like the carbohydrate foods (sugars and starches). When you are eating proteins and fats with the carbohydrates, you have a slower, sustained raise in blood sugar so that you prevent hunger. This is why low-carb diets have been effective at helping people lose weight.

If you are trying to avoid hunger and still lose weight, you want to be aware of how your body reacts to foods so you can make choices that keep your overall glycemic load low enough to prevent blood sugar spikes and with enough protein and fat to keep your blood sugar at a good level so that you feel full (but not stuffed). Notice how you feel after you eat certain foods. Do you find that if you eat sweets, you are soon hungry again? Do you crave more sweets? I found that eating concentrated sweets such as candy, fruit juice, pastries or even gum with sugar would soon result in more hunger and cravings for more sweets. For me, sugar gives me the kind of reaction that is similar to addiction. The more of it I eat, the more I want. I have had others tell me that they have the same kind of reaction to bread. What foods trigger you to want more of them?

For quite a few years now, nutritionists have been telling us to eat low fat diets and during the time that this has been the case, the obesity rate has continued to climb. Many of those so called "diet foods" have lowered the amount of fat but increased the amount of sugar. While eating excessive amounts of fat isn't healthy, fat gives our food flavor and is an energy source that absorbs slowly and helps maintain a stable blood glucose level. Starchy foods such as grains, especially whole grains are recommended as "healthy" and certainly grains make up the largest portion of the American diet. We will talk more about grains in the next chapter.

What about Grains?

There has been a lot of concern recently about gluten and about wheat. The government recommendations show grains and cereals as being the food group that we want to eat the most of and most dieticians follow their guidelines of more than six servings a day. Meanwhile, you see a lot of people following a Paleo diet or the Wheat Belly diet which advocate against the use of grains and reporting that they are losing weight. With all the conflicting information, you may find it difficult to know what to do.

The Paleo diet is based on the idea that our hunter-gatherer ancestors did not farm and grow grains. They ate whatever fruit, vegetable or other plant foods that were available in the area where they lived, fished and hunted wild animals. The sweetener used was wild honey when they could find it. Since they didn't keep livestock, they didn't have access to dairy foods, although they could collect eggs from wild birds. So the diet consists of meat, eggs, fish, vegetables, fruit, nuts and seeds plus a little honey or maple syrup. The Paleo diet is high in protein and fat and low in carbohydrates. There is some debate as to what our ancestors actually did eat since writing had not been developed yet and they didn't leave a record for us. Theoretically, they probably gathered some wild grains but they certainly would not get the quantity of grains that we use in our diets and the wheat grain was different as humans have been breeding it for many years to produce larger kernels and be more productive.

Wheat today is very different than it was even less than 100 years ago. It has been hybridized, that is, bred to have different characteristics. The efforts to hybridize wheat increased during the 1960's and 1970's to produce a wheat that was shorter and had larger seeds. Because food production has been industrialized, our food has been bred, not for health, but to keep well during storage and transportation. In the case of bread, industrial bakers want flour that will rise quickly and produce a light, rather than dense, bread.

What changed in the wheat was a big increase in gluten and gliaden, one of the proteins that make up gluten. Gliaden is the component of wheat that has been linked to a number of diseases and is also considered an appetite stimulant, according to Dr. William Davis, author of the bestselling book, *Wheat Belly.* Gluten helps bread rise and makes the dough stretchy and moldable. The hybridization of wheat has also increased the amount and type of wheat germ agglutinin, a substance that the wheat plant uses to protect itself from insects and molds. This substance is not broken down during the digestive process but can pass through the intestinal wall, acting on insulin to increase fat storage, causing immune problems such as rheumatoid arthritis and worsening, or possibly even causing, celiac disease. Celiac disease is the most severe form of gluten intolerance. If you have either a full blown case of severe celiac disease or an allergic reaction to wheat, you are probably already avoiding it. But many people with gluten sensitivity or less severe cases of celiac disease are unaware they have it.

What about those who are unaware of any problems with gluten? Well, some studies have shown that people consume about 418 less calories per day when wheat is removed from their diet. That would be 2926 less calories per week. To lose a pound of body weight, you generally have to cut back by 3500 calories so just removing wheat from your diet could lead to the loss of a little less than a pound a week or about 43 pounds a year. Dr. Davis has also linked wheat to abdominal fat, elevated blood sugar, acid reflux, bowel urgency, joint pain, leg swelling, migraine headaches, skin rashes, dandruff, moodiness, sleeplessness, depression, seizures and dementia to name just some of the disorders. If you check the glycemic index, you will notice that white bread and your average whole wheat bread are quite high. In fact, a Snickers candy bar has a lower number on the glycemic index. A recent study by researchers in Brazil has confirmed the role of gluten in weight gain, regardless of calorie intake.

I had tried elimination diets and was never able to identify a reaction to any foods. However, when I eliminated wheat and cut back on sugar, my food cravings stopped, my asthma disappeared and I lost weight. My blood sugar improved and I felt better. I am not gluten free because I do eat some grains such as oats, barley (which contain gluten), millet and rice. I do limit the amounts and try to not exceed three servings a day. Gluten free products must be used with caution as many of them contain substances that may be high on the glycemic index.

Sweeteners

We have already talked about sugary foods raising blood sugar, which causes the release of insulin so that blood sugar drops as the glucose is moved into the cells where it may be stored as fat. There is actually something worse than sugary foods and that is sugary drinks. You can take in an amazing amount of sugar very quickly by drinking things with sugar and many people get the majority of the sugar in their diet this way. Did you know that 12 oz of a typical soft drink contains the equivalent of 10 teaspoons of sugar? If you are drinking a 32 oz container you are getting almost three times that much! Not only that, but it is probably in the form of high fructose corn syrup which is actually considered to be worse than sugar.

Fruit juice is also high in sugar. Twelve ounces of orange juice contains about the same amount of sugar as a soft drink. So, even though we think of juice as a "natural" food, it can contribute to a high sugar intake. When you eat an orange or an apple, you generally only eat one piece of fruit. When you make juice, you use multiple pieces of fruit to make one glass of juice. You get all the sugar from the fruit and what you are losing is the fiber, the part that helps you feel full and that slows absorption.

Sugar is added to many of our foods today and in foods that have a lot of it, the food manufacturers will hide it by using several different kinds of sugar under different names. This means that sugar doesn't appear as the first ingredient in foods such as breakfast cereals, even though it might be the most common ingredient. Instead of "sugar", the ingredient list might have brown sugar, corn sweetener, corn syrup, dextrose, fructose, fruit-juice concentrate, glucose, high-fructose corn syrup (HFCS), honey, invert sugar, lactose, maltose, malt syrup, molasses, raw sugar, sucrose (which is table sugar) or other types of syrup. These are all sugars.

So what if you are using artificial sweeteners instead of sugar? You would think that would solve the problem, right? Unfortunately, research shows that the use of artificial sweeteners tends to increase appetite and leads to weight gain. The more artificial sweetener used, the higher the BMI. Diet sodas have been linked to an increased risk of developing diabetes.

There is a lot of controversy regarding artificial sweeteners. The FDA says that they are safe but there are studies that indicate that they are not completely safe. I'll take all of the sweeteners besides the sugars and give you some information about each so you can make a better decision as to what to use.

Sugar alcohols

These are not sugars or alcohols but have a chemical structure similar to sugar and alcohol which gave them this name. They are found in some foods that are labeled sugar-free such as candies, gum, jelly, frozen foods and baked goods. They are easy to recognize on food labels because they generally end in "tol". They do have calories but less than sugar and are not absorbed completely so that they do not raise blood sugar quickly like the sugars do. They also do not contribute to tooth decay. Because of not being completely absorbed, the use of excessive amounts can lead to abdominal gas and diarrhea. Here are the common ones:

- Sorbitol: 2.6 cal/gram and 50% to 70% as sweet as sugar

- Mannitol: 1.6 cal/gram and 50% to 70% as sweet as sugar

- Xylitol: 2.4 cal/gram and 100% as sweet as sugar

- Erythritol: 0.2 cal/gram and 60% to 80% as sweet as sugar

- Isomalt: 2 cal/gram and 45% to 65% as sweet as sugar

- Lactitol: 2 cal/gram and 30% to 40% as sweet as sugar

- Hydrogenated starch hydrolysates: 3 cal/gram and 25% to 50% as sweet as sugar

- Maititol: 2.1 cal/gram and 90% as sweet as sugar.

Stevia

Rebana is the sweet substance found in the Stevia leaf. It is many times sweeter than sugar but has no calories and no effect on blood sugar. Unfortunately, it does have a bitter aftertaste. It is sometimes mixed with other substances because of this. Truvia is a mix of stevia and erythritol. Sweet Leaf is a mix of stevia and inulin, a soluble fiber.

Saccharin

The brand names for saccharin are Sweet and Low, Sweet'N Low, Sweet Twin and Necta Sweet. It has been around for a long time so more research has been done on it. At one time a ban was proposed because it was found to cause bladder tumors in rats. Since it was the only available artificial sweetener at that time, there was a public outcry and Congress decided to allow it in the food supply with a warning label. Human studies, which used lower amounts per body weight than that given to the rats, did not result in cancer and the warning labels were removed. It could possibly be a weak carcinogen. Because it is in the class of sulfonamides, it could potentially cause an allergic reaction in people who are allergic to sulfa drugs. It has a bitter aftertaste.

Aspartame

Also known as Nutrasweet, Equal, Amino Sweet and Sugar Twin, aspartame was approved by the FDA in 1981 and has been approved in over 100 countries. It is now found in many foods including diet sodas. It is one of the most controversial artificial sweeteners and has been linked to a number of negative health effects. Headaches are one of the most commonly reported and it appears that migraine sufferers may have more frequent and more severe migraines with its use. Other problems reportedly linked to aspartame include depression, changes in vision, changes in heart rate, memory loss, sleep problems, seizures, abdominal problems (including nausea and vomiting), joint pain and cancer. It cannot be used by people with phenylketonuria.

Sucralose

This sweetener was originally developed when researchers were trying to create a new insecticide. It is found in Splenda and is known for being "made from sugar". However it is not like sugar and contains chlorine, which is a carcinogen and toxic. It is not known if it is digested and absorbed and there have been no long term studies on humans. Some of the symptoms that have been reported with its use include intestinal gas, diarrhea, nausea, rashes, hives, itching, wheezing, cough, runny nose, chest pains, anxiety, anger and depression. It may also affect the absorption of medication. Splenda contains dextrose and maltodextrin in addition to sucralose so does have some calories.

Acesulfame K

This sweetener has been approved since 1988 and you may see it on food labels. It may also be called Sunett or Ace-K. It lacks long-term testing and contains a known carcinogen called methylene chloride. This can cause headaches, depression, mental confusion, nausea and may affect the liver and kidneys in addition to causing cancer.

Neotame

This is a new version of aspartame that doesn't contain phenylalanine so can be used by people with phenylketonuria. It is sweeter than aspartame. It is primarily used as a flavor enhancer. There is not enough research to know whether it is safe.

One of the big problems with the calorie free artificial sweeteners is that they are linked to weight gain, rather than weight loss. There have been several studies that show that the more artificial sweetener used, the higher the BMI. It seems that when we consume sweetness without calories, our bodies expect the calories and cause food cravings. In studies, rats given artificial sweeteners ate more calories than those given sugar. In human studies, a sweet taste from either natural or artificial sweeteners appears to increase appetite but those using artificial sweeteners actually gained more weight.

I hope by now that you are reading labels to see what is in your food. If this is a new activity for you, I'm sure you will be surprised by all the added ingredients, including sugars.

Real Food vs. Processed Foods

The more I learn about food, what is in it and the way it is processed, the more particular I get about what I am willing to eat. Once upon a time, our country was filled with small family farms and even those who didn't have a farm probably had a garden unless they lived in an apartment. People knew where their food came from and how it was produced. Most of our food supply today is produced by giant corporations whose goal is to make money. They are not looking out for your health.

I think it is important for people to know as much as possible about food so that they can make good choices. I want to educate you about what you are eating and how it affects you. I find that this helps me to stay motivated to eat well over the long term. What we do over the long term makes all the difference in not only getting the weight off but keeping it off.

Research has shown that **the hormones, antibiotics and pesticides found in our food affect our weight.** Some of these we get from eating animals given these products and others are sprayed on or found in plant foods. We have all kinds of additives in our foods, designed to make them taste better so we will want to eat more of them. The food we are eating today is not the food of our grandparents and this plays a role in why obesity is so prevalent today.

Let's start with meat, fish and poultry. Do you picture animals grazing on a hillside until they are big enough to slaughter? Think again. While this once true, today, animals raised for meat are in CAFOs which stands for Confined Animal Feeding Operations.

Cattle may actually start out on pasture but they are sent to feed lots where they are living in pens full of manure surrounded by feed bins. They are given antibiotics, hormones and other chemicals to make them get fatter. Because they aren't moving around a lot, they tend to put on more fat. This is the marbling that is prized in meat because it makes it tender when you grill or cook it at high temperatures. The feed they are given can contain animal byproducts or basically anything cheap that will help them gain weight. Mad cow disease was spread by cows eating byproducts from other cows that were infected so now they feed them byproducts from other animals besides cows. They are fed grain because this fattens them and makes them taste good.

Cattle have four stomachs because they are designed to eat grass. The four stomachs enable them to break down cellulose and other fibers found in plants that we cannot digest. When they are fed grain, this is actually bad for their health and causes liver damage over time. Their overall poor health plus all the feces that they are carrying with them to the slaughter house from their hooves and legs contribute to the occasional outbreaks of a strain of E coli bacteria that have resulted in deaths of people who ate undercooked hamburger.

Pigs spend their entire lives in warehouses and will probably never even see the sun except during transport to a slaughterhouse. They are kept in small crates where they often exhibit strange behaviors because of not being able to act like pigs. In a sense, it drives them crazy. Pigs are at least as intelligent as dogs and are social animals so this type of life is really difficult for them. They are given antibiotics to keep them from getting sick in this overcrowded environment and also to help fatten them.

Because of our preference for the breast meat of chickens, they have been bred so that the chickens grown for meat can barely walk because of their oversized breasts. They are often debeaked because otherwise they would peck each other due to overcrowding since they are packed into warehouses. The chickens used for eggs have a more normal anatomy but they are still debeaked and kept in cages. What about the "cage-free" eggs? This usually doesn't mean the hens get to go outside and scratch and peck like a normal chicken. This means that they get to be loose in the warehouse. If you have ever seen an egg from a chicken that lives on pasture, you will notice that the egg yolk is almost orange in comparison with the yellow yolks from the warehoused chickens.

The processing of animals for food is another concern but one I am not going to address here since it isn't an issue that affects your weight. You might want to read up on the conditions in slaughterhouses but I warn you. You just might want to become vegetarian or vegan afterward. Or you may start looking for a small, local farmer.

If you read packages of fish, you may notice that some of them say "wild caught" and others don't. The ones that don't say, are probably farmed fish. This means they live in artificial ponds where they can be fed cheap food. Once again, they are not as healthy as wild fish.

All of these systems for confining animals produce lots of waste. You can imagine the feces produced when you crowd animals together. There is often contamination of water supplies near these CAFOs. So, in addition to producing fat, unhealthy animals full of chemicals and the cruelty of overcrowding, you have environmental impacts.

Most animal feed contains genetically modified soy and corn. A genetically modified organism (GMO) is one that is produced in a laboratory by taking genetic material from one organism and inserting it into another. This is nothing like the practice of farmers of breeding a plant or animal with a desirable trait to another with a desirable trait that has gone on for thousands of years. This is an entirely new process where genetic material is taken from a completely different kind of organism in a way that could never occur naturally. In most cases, the new organism, which is patented by the company who developed it, is created to resist certain pests or weed killers. For example, Round-Up Ready soybeans can be sprayed heavily with the weed killer, Round-Up and won't die. The weeds around it will die. Bt corn produces a substance called Bt that will make the stomachs of pests who eat it burst open, killing them. I can't imagine that it is good for us. As the weeds and pests become resistant to the weed and pest killers, the amounts used have increased so we are getting more of these in our food than we ever did in the past.

There are several problems with GMOs. First of all, having these chemicals in our diet can cause ill effects on us. Many of the GMO products in our food are in the form of additives that can affect our weight. The brief studies done by the chemical companies don't prove that they are safe for long term use. Longer studies on animals plus reports from farmers show that animals fed GMOs do suffer health problems. There has been an increase in food allergies in humans since GMOs have been introduced which may be related to their use. The use of Round-Up has been linked to kidney disease and other ailments. Secondly, because the weeds are developing resistance to Round-Up and similar chemicals and increasing larger amounts of the weed killer is needed to control them, these chemicals could become ineffective. Third, the pollen from these patented crops blows into other fields contaminating the normal plants. Monsanto, the company that makes Round-Up and Round-Up ready seeds, has been filing suits against farmers whose fields have been contaminated this way, claiming that the farmers have the patented organism that Monsanto created, even though the farmer doesn't want it. If the farmer is growing organic crops that become contaminated, he will lose his organic certification. Or if he is selling his crop overseas, the country it is going to may reject it because they don't allow GMOs. Most other countries label GMOs if they don't outright ban them. The US and Canada are exceptions.

Our use of pesticides is also causing a problem for bees and butterflies. We need these pollinators to create our fruits, nuts and seeds, and for the propagation of vegetables. If the bees all die off, so will we.

And that leads us to the fruits, vegetables and other foods we eat that come from plants. We are getting a lot more toxic chemicals from our food because of what is sprayed on the GMO crops as well as the pesticides used on other crops. The most common GMO foods are: soy, corn, canola, sugar beets, papaya, yellow crookneck or zucchini squash Foods that are sprayed with a lot of pesticides include apples, celery, cherry tomatoes, cucumbers, grapes, nectarines, peaches, strawberries, spinach, sweet peppers, potatoes, blueberries, lettuce, kale and collard greens. It is safest to eat only organic versions of these. So far, it is safe to buy conventional versions of asparagus, avocado, cantaloupe, cabbage, grapefruit, eggplant, kiwi, onions, peas, pineapple, sweet potatoes watermelon and winter squash. Conventional sweet corn and mangoes can be purchased as long as you know they are not genetically modified versions. By making these changes, you reduce the amount of toxins you receive from your food.

Dairy products should also be organic. Otherwise, the milk will likely contain a hormone called rBGH (bovine growth hormone). Cows who give organic milk are also supposed to have access to pasture instead of living in feed lot type conditions where they are fed genetically modified food.

Even how you store your food makes a difference. Cans are lined with plastic containing BPA, a chemical you want to avoid. Plastic containers may have BPA or other toxic substances that can leach into your food, especially if they are exposed to heat. If you use bottled water (which I don't recommend), make sure the plastic bottles are not exposed to sunlight. If you use a microwave, put your food in glass containers rather than any type of plastic. Chemicals like BPA mimic estrogen and have a negative effect on your efforts to lose weight.

In summary, if you want to avoid chemicals that can cause weight gain and to eat healthy food, buy:

1. grass-fed beef
2. organic, preferably pasture raised, poultry and eggs
3. organic dairy products
4. organic vegetables and fruits if they are ones that have lots of pesticides or are likely to be genetically modified.

5. Glass food containers. Avoid the use of plastics for heating or storing food.

Next let's look at foods that come in boxes and cans and how to read food labels.

What is in that Package?

When you pick up a package of a food that has a picture of a barn and the word "natural" on it, what does that bring to mind? The folks who designed that package want you to think that the food is good for you. What does it actually mean? Nothing. That's right, there is no legal definition for the word "natural" on a food. When I see the word "natural" on a product, I wonder what they are trying to hide.

Reading the food's label is a much better way to judge what you are getting. The most important thing to look at is not the nutrition label but the list of ingredients. These are listed in order of how much of something is in the food, by weight. Remember in the chapter on sweeteners, I told you how manufacturers who want to hide how much sugar is in a product may put in several different kinds of sugar so that each of them will be lower on the list of ingredients. So the ingredient list gives you an idea of how much of something is present.

It will also list things that you probably can't pronounce and may have never heard of. Chances are good that some of those may be additives made from genetically modified soy or corn. At least 70% of our food now has genetically modified ingredients. There may be artificial colors, flavors or flavor enhancers to make the food more appealing to you. There may be some preservatives to give it longer shelf life. There may be additives to give it a better consistency.

Here is a list of additives and ingredients that are probably genetically modified unless they are labeled as organic or non-GMO: aspartame, baking powder, canola oil, caramel color, cellulose, citric acid, cobalamin (vitamin B 12), condensed milk, confectioners sugar, corn flour, corn masa, corn meal, corn oil, corn sugar, corn syrup, cornstarch, cotton seed oil, cyclodextrin cysteine, dextrin, dextrose, diacetyl, diglyceride, erythritol, Equal, food starch, fructose, glucose, glutamate, glutamic acid, glycerides, glycerin, glycerol, glycerol monooleate, glycine, hemicellulose, high fructose corn syrup (HFCS), hydrogenated starch, hydrolyzed vegetable protein, inositol, inverse syrup, inversol, invert sugar, isoflavones, lactic acid, lecithin, leucine, lysine, malitol, malt, malt syrup, malt extract, maltodextrin, maltose, mannitol, methylcellulose, milk powder, milo starch, modified food starch, modified starch, mono and diglycerides, monosodium glutamate (MSG), Nutrasweet, oleic acid, phenylalanime, phytic acid, protein isolate, sorbitol, soy flour, soy isolates, soy lecithin, soy milk, soy oil, soy protein, soy protein isolate, soy sauce, starch, stearic acid, sugar (unless it specifically states that it is cane sugar), tamari, tempeh, teriyaki marinades, textured vegetable protein, threonine, tocopherols (vitamin E), tofu, triglyceride, vegetable fat, vegetable oil, whey, whey powder and xanthan gum.

One of the things I always look at is what kind of fats and oils are present. There has been a lot of research to show that "trans-fats" are not good for us. These are oils that have been partially or completely hydrogenated to make them more solid and stable at room temperatures. This is great for the shelf life of the food but not good for the person who eats it. At one time, we were taught that margarine was healthier than butter. Margarine is hydrogenated and we have since discovered that it is not healthy at all. This is also true of shortening such as Crisco, which we once thought was healthier than lard. When you read the nutrition label, a food may say it has no trans-fats but when you see partially hydrogenated vegetable oil on the label, it does. It turns out that as long as the amount of trans-fats is below a certain level, the food can say it doesn't have trans-fats when it actually does. Canola (also known as rapeseed), corn, cottonseed and soybean oils are most likely genetically modified. Many other vegetable oils are heated at high temperatures as part of their processing so that they are unhealthy. The production of palm oil has resulted in clearing of jungle areas that are necessary habitat for endangered species so should be avoided.

Monounsaturated oils are recommended as healthy. Olive oil is a good monounsaturated oil but cannot be used for cooking at higher temperatures such as frying. Coconut oil works well for that. Avocado oil is very good. I also use organic butter. Saturated fat found in meats and dairy has been vilified for a number of years but the most recent research shows that while it doesn't improve health, it doesn't harm it either, which considering how conventional meat and dairy are raised, is saying a lot. The fats found in grass-fed beef are much healthier than those in conventional beef. Fat gives taste and a good texture to food and keeps us full longer. Even though it has more calories per gram than proteins and carbohydrates, healthy fat in moderate amounts can help you lose weight.

The easiest way to avoid all kinds of additives in your food is to make it yourself from healthy ingredients. If you don't know how to cook, it is worth learning and really isn't all that difficult. There are lots of foods that are easy to prepare and while it takes a bit more effort than heating a frozen meal in the microwave, you are getting a much healthier meal.

So What Should I Eat?

Now that you have learned a lot about food, it is time to talk about how to eat in a way that will help you to lose weight, that is, how to apply what you have learned. I don't count calories, don't write down what I eat and generally eat three meals a day, with occasional snacks if I get hungry (which isn't often). If you want to write down what you eat, that's fine but I find it to be too much bother.

Think about how thin people eat. Usually, they eat when they are hungry, stop eating when they stop being hungry and don't obsess about food. Since what you are doing is changing your approach to food and eating as a permanent thing, forget the "going on a diet" mindset. Think about changing habits instead. Changing a habit may make you feel good for the first day or two but is usually uncomfortable for the first couple of weeks. Depending on what the habit is and how well established other habits you have which may be in conflict with the new habit, the first week or so may be awful but if you stick with it, it gets easier. You want to commit to the new habit or habits for at least 60 days. If you make it that far, you will have the new habit established.

With that being said, here is what I eat:

- Lot of vegetables, mostly organic except for the low pesticide, non-GMO ones.
- Whole fruit, organic or conventional depending on pesticide use
- Organic eggs, pastured if possible
- Organic dairy including milk, butter, cheese, sour cream, cottage cheese etc.
- Grass-fed beef
- Organic poultry
- Wild caught fish
- Non-GMO xylitol for sweetening. I sometimes use Stevia with inulin also.
- Nuts and seeds (preferably raw) and almond butter
- Beans
- Quinoa
- Olive oil and coconut oil
- Coconut flour and almond flour for baking
- Some gluten-free bread (read labels) because it is easier than making it.

- Occasional nitrite-free bacon and hot dogs (organic, grass-fed beef)
- Old fashioned oats, barley, brown rice and gluten-free pasta made from brown rice
- Sea salt and mostly organic herbs and spices
- Organic, fair-trade coffee and tea

I started by cutting out sugar as much as possible and once I was comfortable with that I eliminated wheat. Don't be surprised if you crave both of these when you first remove them from your diet. The cravings are normal and temporary, so just hang in there. I went through my cupboards and removed anything that had wheat or significant amounts of sugar. All the unopened packages went to the food bank and the rest went in the trash. It is a lot easier to avoid temptation if you don't allow it into the house. I got wheat-free cookbooks and ingredients used in wheat-free recipes. I don't do much baking but it is good to have a resource if I decide I want to make something.

I don't eat soy because I developed an allergy to it when I was vegan and using quite a bit of it. If you want to eat soy, buy organic, fermented products. Unfermented soy has phytic acid which isn't good for you. Soy also has estrogenic properties which can contribute to weight gain. I suspect that the soy allergy and wheat were the reasons that I not only could not lose weight as a vegan but actually gained.

I don't eat fruit or high glycemic foods unless I have some form of protein and/or fat with them. I enjoy a piece of fruit at the end of a meal but if I want a snack between meals, I am more likely to eat a dozen almonds or a small piece of cheese.

I enjoy drinking coffee first thing in the morning with some milk or half and half. The rest of the day, my most common beverage is plain, filtered, tap water. I also drink green tea, oolong tea or herbal tea. If you live in an area where you have fluoridated water, you will want to have reverse-osmosis filtering to remove it. The fluoride added to water supplies has ill effects on the body including the thyroid gland.

In addition to eliminating wheat and avoiding sugar, I avoid factory farmed meat and genetically modified foods. This means shopping somewhere other than your traditional grocery store. Do you have a farmer's market in your area? Most places have at least one and sometimes several of them. This is a great place to get vegetables, fruit and sometimes, meat and eggs. Alternate grocery stores such as Whole Foods have lots of organic products, grass-fed beef etc. If you have local farms, you may be able to find one that has pastured meat and eggs or organic produce. Some farms offer CSAs (community supported agriculture) where you pay an annual fee and get a box of whatever they produce from them throughout the growing season.

If you have a yard or even a place to put containers, you can grow your own food. I grow tomatoes, peppers and herbs in containers. I compost vegetable and fruit scraps (peels, cores or whatever) and mix that into my potting soil before planting each year. Growing your own is almost like getting free food and helps offset the higher prices for the healthy food you are buying. Having a few hens for eggs is relatively easy to do if it is allowed in your area.

As I mentioned before, I cook most of my food from scratch with fresh ingredients. This gives me the advantage of knowing exactly what is in my food and avoiding additives. I use plenty of herbs and spices for lots of flavor. Herbs are also a great source of nutrients and antioxidants.

A typical day might look like this:

Breakfast:

    Coffee with half and half

    Two eggs cooked in butter

Lunch:

    ¾ cup of cottage cheese

    A large bowl of vegetable soup

Mid-afternoon snack:

    A handful of almonds

Dinner:

    Organic chicken thighs sautéed with a little coconut oil and seasoned with curry powder

    1 to-2 cups of steamed broccoli with butter

    Maybe a little of the brown rice I fixed for my spouse

    An apple for dessert

I don't have any rigid formula for what I eat. I've noticed that I do better with a high protein breakfast. Today, I fixed oatmeal but added whey protein to the cold water before heating it and then added old fashioned rolled oats, nuts, dried fruit, xylitol and vanilla. I eat some protein with each meal whether it is animal protein or plant protein from foods like beans and nuts. Some days I eat more starchy foods than others. It just depends on what I feel like eating and what is on hand. I don't count or measure anything. Eating like this is not a struggle. I don't have food cravings and I eat things I enjoy. If I want pancakes for breakfast, I can make them with alternative flours like almond flour and coconut flour. I'll have eggs with them to make sure I get plenty of protein.

When you are fixing food for other people, you have to take their needs into consideration as well. My husband eats more than I do and he wants more carbs in his diet so I fix pasta, potatoes, rice, pancakes, French toast, etc. for him. Sometimes I eat these and sometimes not. When I fixed stroganoff this week, he had his over rice pasta and I had mine over broccoli. When I made lasagna, I had layers of zucchini along with the rice lasagna noodles, meat, cheese and sauce so I ate the noodles but got extra veggies.

I think about making healthy choices rather than calories but also about what is in season and what I like.

You should only pick foods that you like. Don't ever force yourself to eat foods you hate because they are healthy. Kale is a healthy food but I don't like the taste of it so I don't eat it. I would rather eat other leafy greens that I like, such as spinach. There are such a wide variety of foods to choose from that there is no reason to eat foods you don't like.

If you have not been one to eat vegetables in the past, do some experimentation and try different ones. Look for recipes that use different vegetables. One of the interesting things about being in a CSA is that you will probably get some things you have never tried before and some CSAs will even give you some recipes for using them. Chances are that you will find some that you like, especially if you know how to fix them.

Grass-fed beef or meat from wild animals such as deer, have less fat and marbling than conventional meat. With ground meat, this might not make much difference but if you are fixing a grass-fed steak, don't expect to throw it on the grill and have it come out tender. It needs to be cooked at a lower temperature. The same steak sautéed on low heat with a cover will turn out much better. You could also marinate it and cook it slowly over a cooler fire on the grill.

I don't go out to eat a lot simply because it is more difficult to get what I want. Generally, if you tell your server about what you want (and don't want), they can help you find some reasonably good choices. Some restaurants have "allergy menus" that can be helpful. Ordering simple foods without sauces or added ingredients helps you avoid things you don't want. Don't be afraid to ask questions and to ask for substitutions. There are lot of people who have gone gluten-free so finding wheat-free products such as pasta is much easier than it used to be. Perhaps eating wheat isn't a problem for you and you can just eat limited amounts of whole grain products but for many people, eating wheat is going to cause food cravings.

If I go out to a restaurant or a friend's house, I'm going to be a lot less picky than I would be when I am eating at home. If I am eating good food most of the time, occasional lapses in that aren't going to be an issue. I chose to have organic ice cream on my husband's birthday but not cake. I stick with no wheat or soy all the time because my body doesn't tolerate them and am flexible about the other things. Overall, I am getting far less GMOs, pesticides, hormones and antibiotics in my food.

One more thing that it is important to mention is that you want to get plenty of water to drink. Sometimes people think they are hungry when they are really thirsty. If you haven't developed the habit of drinking water, this is a good time to start. If you really don't like water, try some herbal tea. I occasionally add some lemon juice and xylitol to my water to make lemonade but most of the time, I just drink plain cold water (I keep a pitcher in the fridge) and sip it all day long while I am working.

Exercise

I have had kind of a love-hate relationship with exercise. I am not one of those people who wakes up in the morning and says "I can't wait to go exercise". I have a habit of doing it and I feel really good about having done it. I like being able to see and feel muscles giving my body a better shape. But I can't say I get excited about doing it and am not one of those people who wants to do triathlons or marathons. I have tried running in the past but my knees don't like it. I have gone to gyms but it is not convenient. I have a program that is easy, I can do at home and where I do the least amount of exercise for the most benefit. It takes me about 15 minutes per day. Even though it is now a habit, I still have days where I have to push myself to do it. One thing I can say is that it feels way better than it did when I was heavier. It was hard work, lugging that extra weight around and it is no wonder that most people who are overweight don't enjoy exercise.

So why exercise? If you are just looking at calories, eating less food has a lot bigger impact than exercise does but that isn't looking at the whole picture. Exercise speeds up your metabolism for a few hours after you do it, in addition to the extra calories you burn while you are actually exercising. One of the biggest benefits is that it builds muscle. Muscle burns calories all the time. More muscle means more calories burned...at rest! Women, this is why men lose weight easier than you do. They naturally have more muscle because of having more testosterone and less estrogen. Muscle weighs more than fat so if you are building muscle while losing fat, it won't show on your scale as much as it will in your clothes. If the scale hasn't moved but your clothes are getting loose, you are losing fat. Exercise also strengthens your bones, helps your immune system, improves your endurance so you don't get tired as easily, reduces the risk of chronic diseases like diabetes and heart disease and if you should have a heart attack, you are more likely to survive it. It reduces your risk of cancer, helps with arthritis, raises your HDL (good) cholesterol and reduces your triglycerides. It can improve balance, help you sleep better, reduce blood pressure and is as effective for depression as taking antidepressant medication without the side effects. With all of that going for it, you want to make sure you include it as an important part of your life.

Most exercise falls into two categories, either aerobic or anaerobic. Aerobic means that you are working at an intensity where you are not getting out of breath. Walking is an example of aerobic exercise. Anaerobic exercise means that you are working your muscles at a more intense level such as sprinting or weight lifting so that you can only continue for a shorter period of time. What is aerobic for an experienced exerciser might be anaerobic for a beginner. For best results you want some of each.

One of the best ways to check your intensity level is to check your pulse. You can do this at the thumb side of your inner wrist or at the carotid artery at the side of your neck (only check one side as you don't want to reduce blood flow to the brain). By laying the index and middle fingers gently over the area, you should be able to feel your pulse. This gets easier with practice. Then you count the beats, for either six seconds and add a zero at the end, or count for 15 seconds and multiply by four, to get your heart rate. The 15 second method is more accurate but if you are just looking for a quick estimate, the six second method works.

To calculate your maximum heart rate for exercise, subtract your age from 220.

Subtract your resting heart rate

Multiply by 50% and then separately multiply by 85%.

Take each of these numbers and add your resting heart rate.

For example, if you are 30 years old and have a resting heart rate of 75:

220-30=190.

190-75=115   115x.50=57.5+75=132.5
115x.85=97.75+75=172.75

So this means to exercise in the aerobic range, your pulse should be between 133 and 173.

The usual recommendation for aerobic exercise is at least 20 minutes on at least three days a week. Doing 30 minutes of aerobic exercise five days a week is better if you are working at the lower end of your target range.

Walking fast enough to raise your heart rate into the target zone is a good choice for many people. You should be working at a level where you can carry on a conversation but would be breathing too hard to be able to sing.

I like interval training. This means that you exercise at a higher intensity for a few minutes, slow down a minute to bring your pulse rate down and then speed up the exercise again. This means that you are pushing a bit beyond the typical "aerobic" level. . Because of the bursts of higher intensity exercise, you are burning more calories and you are also conditioning your heart and lungs for better performance and endurance. I am also including exercises that use my body weight to build muscle such as push-ups and lunges. Alternating fast and slow walking or running and walking if that works for you, is also interval training and adding a bit of weight lifting afterward gets you the same results. Warm up by starting with low intensity exercise and cool down afterward the same way If you have any health problems or are older, you want to check with your healthcare provider before starting any exercise program.

If there is some sort of exercise that you enjoy, I would encourage you to do that. If, like me, exercise doesn't appeal to you, you just want to find something that you can do without hating it. You have to push yourself to do it every day until it becomes a habit and then keep doing it every day. The most important thing is to find something you can stick with permanently. You may come up with a plan to do different things on different days for more variety or do similar things every day.

In addition to a regular exercise program, you want to try to get more activity into your day. Do you like going for walks or hiking? Do you enjoy sports (playing them, that is; watching them doesn't count)? Are there times when you could walk or ride a bike instead of driving a car? All that activity helps you to feel good and lose weight faster along with keeping the weight off.

Mental Weight Loss

Most of us focus on the physical part of weight loss, what we eat and exercise. There is another aspect that is just as important and that is the mental part of losing weight. The more primitive parts of our brain encourage us to eat, especially high fat and high sugar foods because these urges were useful when we lived in an environment where food was scarce. It helped us to survive. Now we live in an environment where food is abundant and overeating is a problem that could kill us by giving us diseases that have become common such as diabetes. Fortunately, we have rational parts of the brain that we can use to make better choices. But having a mind-set of scarcity where we tell ourselves to eat that yummy food because it might not be there later, can sabotage us. Crash diets where we deprive ourselves of adequate calories and nutrients will definitely trigger the urge to overeat. This is one of the reasons that we gain back all the weight we lose on that type of diet.

If you give up foods, telling yourself that you can't eat them because it is against the "rules" of the diet you are on, you will probably obsess over them and feel deprived. Before you give up anything, you have to decide if this is something you want to do for yourself. You are not going to deprive yourself. Instead, you are going to give yourself a gift of better food choices because you are worth it! You deserve to have a healthy, fit body. You deserve to be slender. You deserve to nourish yourself with good tasting, healthy food. If this doesn't feel true to you, then we need to do some work on changing the messages you give yourself.

Weight loss should not be a struggle where you have to exert willpower to give up all the foods you love for that less desirable, healthy stuff. Willpower has limited usefulness. It can help you through the first part of changing some habits but it is not going to get you thin and keep you there. You have to see yourself as a thin person and eat accordingly because you WANT to. I eat the way I do because it makes me feel better. I deserve better than to eat junk.

I want you to switch from a lifestyle of eating processed junk into a lifestyle where you love yourself into thinness. You are choosing health and wellness. You are choosing to be able to move more easily. You are choosing to be more attractive. You are choosing to be happy (a state which has nothing to do with a number on a scale).

I'm guessing that you probably don't feel this way already because if you did, you would be at a normal weight and wouldn't be reading this book. We touched on this in the chapter on Readiness to Lose Weight. By now, you have realized that eating comfort foods to try to make yourself feel better has limited usefulness. You feel better very briefly and then beat yourself up for eating something "bad" or for eating too much. Then you feel bad about yourself because you are overweight. This is a vicious cycle that you are going to break.

Let's start with happiness. Happiness is a choice. If you depend on circumstances to make you happy, you will probably have brief periods of happiness but it won't be sustained. Regardless of your circumstances, you can choose to look at the positive things or the negative things in your life. It is the old "Is the glass half full or half empty?" situation. If you look for what is good in your life and feel grateful for that, you will find yourself experiencing happiness. So, why do so many of us focus on the negative? It is a bad habit and one that is reinforced by people around us. Can you unlearn this habit and learn to focus on the positive? Yes, you can! It helps if you can find some positive people to be around but another thing that helps is by taking some time every day to write down things that you are grateful for. You don't need to lose weight to be happy. Start now, today, to look for all the things you can be grateful for. Do you have a roof over your head and food to eat? Do you have friends and family that you love? Do you have a job or skill that you are good at? Do you have hobbies that you enjoy? What about groups or organizations that give meaning to your life?

Are you a worrier? Worry is thinking about what awful things could happen in the future. Most of the things we worry about never happen. In fact, almost none of the awful things we think up actually happen. If they do, we will deal with them but by worrying about future possibilities, you are giving up your happiness in the present moment. Think about now, this moment. Is there anything you need to take care of now? If so, do what you need to do. Then get back to enjoying this moment right now because that is all you really have. Worrying about the future or lamenting the past are exercises in futility. You can't change the past and while you want to plan and prepare for the future, worrying doesn't help. What could you do to add some fun or laughter to this present moment?

Next, let's take a look at your self-image. Chances are that when you were a child, people told you things about yourself. When you are young, you don't have the ability to look at these things rationally and decide whether they were true or not. My mom used to make comments that I was stupid or dumb. I was fortunate that my school did IQ testing and then suddenly, from almost flunking, I was classified as "gifted" so got messages from teachers to counter the previous ones but I felt inadequate because of those early messages. We incorporate those messages into our subconscious and then repeat them back to ourselves as we get older without ever questioning if they are true. What are some of the messages you got from the people around you? What messages do you give yourself?

If you have messages like "I will always be fat", "I can't lose weight" or "I don't deserve to be a normal, thin person" in your head, you are going to have a really hard time losing weight. You need to address those messages. Are they true? Looking at them from a rational adult perspective, you can see that they are not. Sometimes it takes some practice to identify that little voice in your head so you can look at what you tell yourself about various situations and come up with a more rational thought. As you are recognizing the thoughts, you can also look at the behaviors that you do as a result. You can make a choice to do something different so that you get a better outcome. If you do the same things you have always done, you will get the same results you have always gotten in the past. Since that didn't make you thin, your thoughts and behaviors need to change to give you the results you want.

There are a couple of things you can do to help change your thoughts. One is hypnosis. There are recorded messages you can listen to that will do this or you can try individual or group sessions with a hypnotherapist. Another thing that helps is self-affirmations. These are positive messages that you read to yourself daily. Affirmations are written as though you have already achieved what you want. Mentally picture yourself as you want to be. Your brain does not know whether what you see is real or not but it will align your behaviors with your self-image. Here are some examples of self-affirmations:

- I love myself, just the way I am right now
- I enjoy eating healthy foods
- I love the way I feel when I exercise
- I am very healthy
- I lose weight effortlessly to be at my ideal weight

You can use these or write some of your own but I want you to stand in front of a mirror and say these to yourself, looking yourself in the eye. You may feel silly at first but keep at it and it will start to feel more natural and eventually, you will start believing them!

You have probably noticed that beating yourself up about being overweight and hating your body hasn't worked for you. Loving yourself and your body, now, today, before you have lost the weight and treating yourself with kindness are much more effective!

If you are struggling with depression, you may find this harder than most people will. Things that help depression include sunlight and exercise. Outdoor exercise can be as effective as antidepressants. Other ways to combat depression include supplements such as 5-HTP and SAMe. You might want to talk to your healthcare provider about these or if he or she is unfamiliar with them, do some research on your own.

Lifestyle Change

There are some other things you can do to increase your ability to achieve and maintain weight loss and the first one is to get enough sleep. When you don't get enough sleep, your levels of leptin, which signals the brain when you are full, go down and the levels of ghrelin, which is an appetite stimulant, go up. Not surprisingly, studies have shown that sleep deprivation leads to overeating, particularly of high carbohydrate and high calorie foods. So, make it a point to get eight hours of sleep every night.

If you wake up tired after eight hours of sleep, especially if you snore, get checked for sleep apnea. This is a condition where a person actually stops breathing for brief periods of time during sleep. As a result of the constant interruptions of breathing, the person does not get restful sleep. Most people with sleep apnea are obese and many lose weight with treatment.

Have you noticed family and friends attempting to sabotage your new lifestyle? When you stay "no" to a food, do you find people saying "but this is a special occasion, surely you could have some this once" or similar kinds of comments? I tell people I am allergic to soy and wheat but I don't say I'm "on a diet" (although they have certainly noticed that I have lost weight). If I don't want something, I say "No, thank you". I don't explain and if they persist, I just say "no, thank you" again. If they keep it up, I tell them I don't want any. If you say you are on a diet, people will assume that you really do want it and are giving it up because of the "diet". They will argue with you about it. If you say you don't want it, there is no way to argue with that. And in fact, when I choose not to eat something, I actually don't want it. If I did, I would eat it.

Another big problem is chronic stress. When we are stressed our adrenal cortex puts out a hormone called cortisol. Small amounts of cortisol such as the amount that is secreted when we are feeling threatened can be helpful by giving us extra energy (to fight or flee from the threat), less sensitivity to pain and a heightened awareness of what is going on around us. These are useful changes when we are in danger. The problem arises when we are staying in a state where we are stressed. Over time, there is a higher level of cortisol in the bloodstream leading to an increase in abdominal fat, lower immune response, decreases in muscle and bone, sugar imbalances, suppression of thyroid function and impairment of cognitive function. Feeling stressed can also lead to emotional eating.

It is important to realize that stress is not caused by what happens to us so much as by our reaction to it. If you see a poisonous snake, poised to strike, you have a reaction. If you think you see the snake but it is not real, you have the same reaction and your body doesn't know the difference. Some people react more than others. If you are one of those people, learning to control this is very important.

Things that can help you to de-stress include exercise. This is just one more reason that exercise needs to be an important part of your daily routine. Meditation puts you into a calm, relaxed state that reduces stress. It is relatively easy to learn and can be done for 15 to 20 minutes a day with great results. Self-hypnosis, listening to soothing music and sex can all help with stress. You might also want to reduce your intake of caffeine. Letting go of worry and living in the present moment makes life much less stressful.

Journaling and especially writing down what you are grateful for each day helps you to feel more positive and those positive feelings will combat the negative feelings that lead to stress. The daily use of affirmations that we talked about previously also helps with this. Remember that it is important to keep your affirmations positive. If you are fighting against being fat, your mind sees you as fat and will work at keeping you the way you see yourself. See yourself as a thin person and love your body, the way it is. Think of all the great things it does for you. You are able to see, to hear, to taste, to feel pleasant sensations, to think, to move. You have organs that keep you alive without you even having to think about them. You are a magnificently designed organism. Even the ability to eat and digest food so you can use it for energy is amazing. Be grateful to your wonderful body.

Achieving and maintaining a healthy weight is going to happen naturally without any struggle. See this happening in your mind. See yourself as healthy and fit. You are going to naturally want to eat healthy foods that make you feel good. You are going to want to be more active and to exercise every day. You are going to find activities that give you pleasure and that because you feel so much better about yourself and your life, you have no reason to turn to food for comfort. Instead, you notice when you are feeling physical hunger and eat in response to that. Because you are eating lower glycemic foods, you don't get hungry easily. Because you love yourself and your body, you are taking good care of yourself.

I start my day with meditation, positive affirmations, visualization of how I want my life to be (normal weight is just a small part of this), exercise and journaling. I also read things that promote self-development. I'm more focused on my goals than I am about weight and food. I'm grateful for everything in my life including my thinner body. I don't have food cravings and eat moderate amounts of good food. I enjoy what I eat. Sometimes I get busy and forget to eat. Eventually, I will notice that I'm hungry and either fix a meal or have a snack to tide me over until my next meal. I sometimes carry snacks with me so I don't end up in a situation where I am hungry and don't see anything healthy that I want to eat. It is faster and easier to just have something available.

To review what you have learned, you understand that a diet mentality and repeated crash diets will make you fatter, you know about how choosing high glycemic foods can make you hungrier and lead to weight gain and you know what a realistic and healthy weight goal for yourself would be. You have learned a lot about food and how to make healthier food choices. You can read labels and have a better idea what is in packaged foods. You know why exercise is so important and the basics of how to exercise. You know more about chemicals and hormones that affect your weight. You have learned a lot about the emotional and mental aspects of weight loss and why these are as important as what you eat and how you exercise. You have learned how to deal with stress and to make your life happier and more fulfilling. Now, it is a matter of trusting the process.

Making the changes we have discussed will probably lead to some rapid weight loss at first but this will slow down. If you have developed good habits and a commitment to continuing these changes, you will slowly reach your goal. It is important to not have unrealistic expectations. I'm guessing that you didn't go from thin to overweight quickly but that this is a problem you have had for a long time. You are trading attitudes and behaviors of a fat person for the attitudes and behaviors of a thin person and regardless of the number on the scale you see today, this will result in a normal weight over time. Merely losing weight will not change your life. Changing your habits, beliefs and attitudes to those of a thin person will. This is the secret to not only losing weight but staying at your healthy, normal weight permanently.

I want to support you in your new life so you are welcome to subscribe to my free newsletter where I will send you support and encouragement along with additional tips to help you. To sign up go to: www.http://app.getresponse.com/site/loseweightwithout hunger/webform.html?wid=2794204&u=2xjw

Wishing you great success!

References

CDC website: Obesity and Overweight for Professionals

Davis, William: *Wheat Belly: Lose the wheat, lose the weight and find your way back to health.* Rodale 2011.

http://www.alternet.org Americans Are Huge: 5 Surprising Reasons Why We May Be Getting Fatter

http://EzineArticles.com/?expert=Lyn_Smith

http://greensciencepolicy.org/topics/health-environment/

Institute of Responsible Technology website: GMOs

Kroger M, Meister K, Kava R. Low-calorie Sweeteners and Other Sugar Substitutes: A Review of the Safety Issues. Comprehensive Reviews in Food Science and Food Safety. 2006; 5:35-47.

Mayo Clinic Staff, Rev up your workout with interval training

NIH website: What Are the *Health* Risks of Overweight and Obesity?

Robertson, Annabelle. WebMD feature article on Interval Training

Yang, Qing, *Neuroscience 2010*, "Gain Weight by going diet? Artificial sweeteners and the neurobiology of sugar cravings.